A Cosmic Understanding of Disease and Cure

A Cosmic Understanding of Disease and Cure

by

Artimia Arian

TASHIRAT COSMIC LEARNING CENTER
TEPOZTLAN, MEXICO

www.Tashirat.com

A Cosmic Understanding of Disease and Cure

Tashirat Learning Center, Tepoztlan, Mexico

© 2009, 2014 by Artimia Arian
All rights reserved*

For information address:
www.Tashirat.com

tashiratmail@gmail.com

The medical and health procedures in this book are based on the research, training and personal experience of the author. As each one of us and each situation is unique, the reader is urged to check with a qualified health professional when in doubt, before applying any procedure, and preferably to work under his / her supervision.

ISBN: 978-1-304-63158-9 (Pbk)

Front & Back Cover Photos by Thyesha Arian

Note to the Reader

This book is replete with knowledge that takes the reader's cosmic consciousness for granted. In addition, it can only be understood if the following books by Artimia Arian are read in the order presented:

Cosmic Reawakening

Vibrational Nutrition

A Cosmic Understanding of Disease and Cure

Timeless Spiritual Teachings

Inspirational Quotes for the New Era

Essential Teachings for the New Era

Spiritual Vision for the New Era

For supplemental information please also read:

To Life!

Chakra Recipe Guide

The Tashirat Recipe Manual

For convenience, the masculine has been utilized not the feminine and they have not been used alternately as was done in some of my other books. No preference of sex is intended.

In Truth, Love and Life,
Artimia Arian

Table of Contents

Introduction

When man's will was united to the Divine Father's, sickness did not exist. But the God of the All needed man to evolve, so he gave him the gift of free will and this gift coincided with the negative kundalini cycle in the Cosmos. Unfortunately, too few possessed purity of heart and so mankind descended into negative emotions of ego, greed, jealousy, vanity and hunger for power and recognition. With these emotions, the evil of wars began and man has experienced the effects of excessive negativity – evil.

The pendulum will swing, because the Cosmic Order is perfect and reigns supreme. Divine Justice is infallible. The New Era, due to the Cosmic Law of Rhythm, will be as excessively positive as the era we are only just emerging from, has been evil. However, evil weakened everybody – the aggressors and the victims alike and now in these transition years leading up to the New Era, we have to begin the clean-up job of purifying and strengthening humanity again.

Hopefully the memory of such disastrous evil will live in our memories forever, so such atrocities never recur. With free will, there are only two paths one can choose from – the Path of Love, Light (Knowledge) and Life and the Path of Darkness and Death.

The Cosmos is vast and consists of zillions of worlds but there are only three types of worlds that exist – positive worlds, negative worlds and neutral worlds. There are many different levels of each of these categories but basically these are the only categories that exist. It is the value system that distinguishes the different category worlds.

Positive worlds focus on serving the God of the All; learning to connect and lead a spiritual life; and on love and knowledge. They focus mostly on medicine and healing and the sciences. Negative worlds focus on money and possessions, power, position and vanity. Positive world people are deeply feeling and conscious, they are only interested in purifying and strengthening themselves in their lives and serving others, their world and their universe. The more one loves and the more knowledge one has, the stronger one gets. Positive world people have very few children but their children are their treasures, their everything.

Negative world people have no feelings as they have lost their hearts through all they have done with impure hearts and they are now numbed to feelings. They are cold and hard and out for themselves and their personal advancement. They are vain, power and recognition hungry and they provoke killing and so much sufferance. They have very many children, who are not that well cared for and who are used to attain their goals of attaining more territory or power.

Neutral world people are highly critical of everything and everyone. They are the non-committal types who have no long-term life goals. They live from day to day, wanting no problems, no wars, and no loyalties that would bind them.

The energies in the Cosmos are swinging slowly positive again, so naturally humanity will start having more emotional, mental and spiritual yearnings. This book is an attempt to demonstrate the origin of disease, as the Earth abounds in chronic degenerative diseases today, that according to orthodox medicine are incurable. If you understand the origin of an imbalance, which is all any disease really is, then you can recreate a balance and bring about a healing.

The Origin of Disease

When man's will was united to God's, before he was given the gift of free will, there was no sickness. This long negative era from which we are finally emerging, was the first time that man had been given free will and he created a disaster. With the gift of free will, man began his descent and he descended so far, that the majority of people in the Cosmos' consciousness waned as they steeped themselves more and more in a physical-oriented materialistic lifestyle, devoid of spirituality and love. The acquisition of possessions, self-aggrandizement, the need for recognition and adoration, physical appearance and the desire to impress others, all forms of manipulation and deceit to seize the power, greed and hunger for power and territory, became all-consuming, all-important.

Before the gift of free will, man's will was united to the God of the All's because he had the consciousness and humility to recognize God's greatness, to love Him with his life and to appreciate and follow His guidance. Man was whole, sickness did not exist. With the gift of free will, man has lived unguided, losing force with wrong thinking and inverted lifestyle habits.

There is light, the positive (not good) and darkness, the negative (not bad). The darkness was created to enhance the light, to strengthen it, to foster evolution. The darkness is the light's shadow; without the light it has no existence of its own. Light dispels darkness but darkness has no power of its own; darkness cannot extinguish the light as it is only light's shadow. In a dark room, if you turn on the light, the darkness disappears. In a room full of light, darkness cannot be turned on, the source of the light has to be blocked or diverted, for the light to disappear from the room. Both the positive and negative energies are a necessity for creation; the ongoing tension between these energies within the individual, between the two sexes, and on a cosmic scale, engenders health, balance, and evolution.

Evil, on the other hand, in the medical or any other context, is imbalance, which is sickness. Evil was the starting point of our destruction, the cause of suffering. With free will, evil, which is excessive negativity, pervaded the Cosmos. What we are living today, is the aftermath. The Positive Era will be brought about by man's consciousness change, which begins with each individual.

Sickness is delusion, a false perception of oneself and reality. A delusion is nothing but a false perception of reality. Disease is a false perception of the present. A perfectly healthy, balanced person is a rarity today, if one such person even exists. Most people live in a physical, emotional, mental or spiritual state of imbalance. This imbalance can be rectified if it is first well understood.

Each person's delusion (disease) can be traced back to his past, to a real life situation in which he employed a survival mechanism appropriate to the situation. He may have been in a terrifying situation and as a survival mechanism, shut down, turned within, and became highly unaware of what he or anyone else was thinking or living. Another survival mechanism could have been to inflict the pain he felt on others who were weaker, in a response to his rage and despair. He may have switched off emotionally and lost all love and passion for life. Whatever survival mechanism was utilized and functioned in the original situation, enabling him to survive, is no longer appropriate in the present, as the situation has changed. However, if this survival mechanism became so deeply ingrained in his mind programming that it determines all of his behavioral responses, controlling his entire life, even though the original situation is no longer present, we have a state of disease or imbalance.

Our feelings, actions and reactions correlate with our deepest beliefs, so many of them highly illogical and existing on a subconscious level. These same beliefs, if extracted and exposed to the conscious mind, can be traced back to their origin – a situation in this life time, a previous Earth life or usually a cosmic life from the second dimension (Earth is the third dimension). These beliefs are but a manifestation of the delusion. Hence to alter dysfunctional mind programming, the delusion(s) that impede you from seeing reality, have to be shattered. The state of body and mind are always related, so the delusions are reflected in both the physical body and the mind. Connections between the body and the mind can be witnessed. For example a person who is rigid in his ideas and manner, may suffer from arthritis or could develop hard nodules, indurations.

Man is healthy because on the second dimension, in his cosmic life, before descending to his third dimensional Earth life, he was not tainted with ego and /or an impure heart, and he has a knowledge of who he is (his cosmic origins) and therefore how he must live his life (for his level of consciousness and vibration). Or man is unhealthy because on the second dimension, in his cosmic life, his consciousness was tainted by ego or impure intentions or because he lacks the knowledge of who he is (his cosmic history) and lacks the knowledge of how to live his life (for his particular evolution i.e. his vibration or consciousness). It is our innermost consciousness (which is often diseased) which leads to manifested symptoms, such as nervousness, feelings of guilt, feelings of apprehension, and all physical symptoms.

We all proceed from the God of the All, the most positive, divine force, but so many people broke their connection to this divinity through their own free-will, which was given and now will never be denied us. Through this severance with their connection to their Father, they continued to plummet in consciousness and lose force. In order for a cure to take place, you have to find your way back to your initial error. Actually we are all part of the Cosmos and its Laws and even the emotional and spiritual break from God, will push you to one day return to Him, because perfect order prevails in the Divine Cosmic Plan of which we are all a part. Although the severance led you in another direction, after suffering enough, you will learn, and by energetic law, you will return to Him.

However, by emotionally breaking with God (heart is everything), the continual influx of God's love and guidance, His protection, is denied you by energetic law too, a law that you set in motion. Water can be pouring into a glass (God's energy, love, protection are always there, He wants to give it all) but if the glass if full (of ego and ego desires and therefore no love for others which would cause the water to flow out and empty the glass), the water just overflows and flows into other glasses that are receptive, being ego empty.

Order is the nature of the Divine Plan. By preserving and cherishing your connection to your Source, you insure order and therefore harmony and happiness in your life. When this connection is broken, disharmony, sickness (energetic imbalances) and suffering ensue on an individual level. This individual disharmony contaminates the energetic ocean to which we are all connected. If too many individuals are out of kilt, as is the case today, even healthier people are affected by the energetic ocean.

We are all connected energetically. Even a stone vibrates with energy, the atoms that comprise it. A stone responds far less than a plant, which responds less than an animal, but the stone does have an intelligent ordering energy, although it does not possess free will or consciousness. A higher more evolved animal exhibits the beginnings of consciousness. The more evolved the animal, the higher the consciousness. Some men's lives are so deeply entrenched and polluted by their lower desires and selfish or evil motives, that their behavior is perverted and their consciousness is actually lower than that of many animals, who are even still controlled by instinct, the subconscious and not conscious mind. We are all connected to everything in creation energetically. However, man has free will, and although Nature portrays a miraculous harmony, man, because of his free will, has the ability to destroy his own harmony, the harmony of his vital force (generating his one illnesses), and that of his environment, thereby affecting people positively or negatively.

The key to disease and therefore cure is in the finer world of cause. No pathology can be divorced from the sickness of the soul and this in turn can be seen in the energetic imbalance of the vital force. It follows that no part of the body can be considered diseased, the whole man is diseased always and needs to be cured. The soul sickness which the vital force clearly manifests in symptoms, be they mental, emotional or physical, must be cured in order for a permanent cure to take place. You cannot isolate and try and cure the symptoms, for example, the malignant tumors or purulent ulcers. The original cause of the energetic imbalance, the soul sickness, has to be dealt with.

Separation from God, for whatever reason, is the root of soul sickness. Connection to God is the soul's healing. There exists no other healing. The deeper the love connection, the greater the healing and the more permanent the cure, as evolution ensues rather than involution. Strength is engendered if the guidance from the connection is obeyed and executed. Weakness in any form is the result of the severance of the connection with the Source. The longer the severance, the more centripetal (selfish) the energies, the greater the resulting debility.

Understanding Disease

According to all medicine – orthodox or alternative – a disease is a syndrome of symptoms that we recognize by virtue of a certain kind of pathology. But in reality, this is but the manifestation of the soul sickness. Depending on the intensity of the disease, if the manifestation affects the physical level, it is less profound and debilitating than if it affects the deeper emotional level. If it affects the mental level, it is the most severe and difficult to heal. But the true cause of disease is a lack of consciousness, which moves from center (consciousness) to circumference. Only a lowered consciousness can cause disease.

Homeopaths define health as a state of freedom of the three bodies – the physical, emotional and mental bodies. A physically healthy person experiences physical vitality, and freedom from physiological malfunction. An emotionally healthy person lives with an inner sense of freedom, harmony and happiness. They don't feel bound. They are outgoing, they feel, comprehend and love people and are natural, free and spontaneous in the expression of their thoughts and feelings. They are not self-centered so they experience the joy of living for others and loving others. Their lives are replete with love. A mentally healthy person does not live in a mental fog. They possess clarity of thought and creativity of thought. The more clear and essence a person is in their written and verbal expression, the stronger the mental body.

First functional disturbances of the vital force will be evident in a person, for example, insomnia, excessive thirst, hypersensitivity to noise, temperature, etc. When the vital force can no longer cope, the imbalance is localized in the least important organ and if that is suppressed or overburdened, it moves to more vital organs. When these organs can no longer cope, it moves out of the physical body realm to the more serious and deeper emotional, mental and spiritual bodies.

Actually the vital force's manifestation will always be targeted to the least important part of the organism when possible, thus preserving the integrity of the whole, but it always manifests in the weakest body, be it physical, emotional or mental, and the weakest part of the body.

"I feel" are functional changes – in the activities of the body, changes in sensations, changes in functions. They precede structural pathological tissue changes. The functional changes appearing as symptoms are a warning. They must be read and dealt with appropriately before further structural changes occur. They reveal the state of disorder that must be rectified before further disorder runs its natural course. If the disorder is not checked, the involution will lead to destruction. The involution is occurring on a deeper plane than merely the physical plane. It is the energy of the person, the vital force, that is unbalanced and must be corrected before it results in pathology in the physical body and moves even deeper into the emotional and mental bodies.

When a treatment is administered correctly, symptoms on the deeper levels improve while those on more external levels are often exacerbated temporarily. The cure can be expected to progress from inside out, and this progress can be used to validate the success of the treatment. There are three general principles of the healing process that were codified by a homeopath, Constantine Hering, that are known as the Laws of Cure. Hering was a German homeopath who emigrated to the United States in the 1830s and is considered the father of American homeopathy. It is important to understand these laws in order to assess the progress of symptoms accurately. Is the treatment successful when a skin ailment disappears or was the ailment suppressed and will it now affect a more vital organ?

According to the first of Hering's laws, healing progresses from the deepest part of the organism – the mental and emotional levels and the vital organs – to the external parts; such as the skin and extremities. A cure is considered successful then, if a person's psychological symptoms improve, even if the physical symptoms increase (as long as the physical symptoms are not severely pathological). Eventually all symptoms must disappear. Beware if the person's physical symptoms improve but their psychological symptoms increase. This means that the person's health is deteriorating.

George Vithoulkas, a contemporary homeopath, has outlined the varying depths of symptoms of each body, in descending order of depth, symptoms and their impact on one's state of health. The exact location of these symptoms in the table is not as important as the outline's use as a guide for evaluating the patient's progress, according to Hering's first law.

Physical	Emotional	Mental
Brain ailments	Suicidal depression	Complete confusion
Heart ailments	Apathy	Destructive delirium
Endocrine ailments	Sadness	Paranoid ideas
Liver ailments	Anguish	Delusions
Lung ailments	Phobias	Lethargy
Kidney ailments	Anxiety	Dullness
Bone ailments	Irritability	Lack of concentration
Muscle ailments	Dissatisfaction	Forgetfulness
Skin ailments		Absentmindedness

Hering's second law states that as healing progresses, symptoms appear and disappear in the reverse of their original chronological order of appearance. It is common for chronic patients to re-experience symptoms from past conditions. They could have suffered from these conditions recently or as many as twenty years ago.

Hering's third law states that the healing progresses from the upper to the lower parts of the body. So if a skin rash from German measles is moving from the neck to the chest, the cure is taking place.

It is important to know that a patient's symptoms may not always conform exactly to these laws. The symptoms may move from within outward, in accordance with the first law, but may also move upward, violating the third law. Whenever the progress of healing is difficult to interpret, the final judgment depends on whether the person experiences an overall increase in freedom and a general improved sense of well- being. An apparent violation of one law may be insignificant if the symptoms that arise are minor. It is most important that the other laws are observed and the person's general state improves (feeling more positive, sleeping better, better appetite, sexual drive, etc.) Hering's Laws are not only used by homeopaths, they are used by acupuncturists, psychotherapists and other healers. It is very important to consider the changes in symptoms in relation to Hering's Laws.

Life in its fullest sense is freedom. Ironically, the severance of man's will from that of God's which was thought to endow him with freedom, actually enslaved him. Without God's guidance, he fell into the snare of ego – his own blinding ego importance (he no longer has the eyes of the Spirit to recognize greatness) and sense pleasures. Living for himself and divulging in the pleasures of the senses, his consciousness became beclouded and dull. He is now enslaved by the senses and lacks the soul consciousness (a strong healthy spiritual body), therefore the will (emotional body – they are always intimately connected), to return to God by once again uniting his will go to God's. If life in its fullest sense is freedom, this enslavement to the senses, resulting from a severance with a positive constructive life as guided by God, is death, emotionally, and ultimately physically and even spiritually. Liberating oneself from sense pleasures is the highest form of self-discipline and therefore liberation, leading one to a far higher quality life, enabling you to be a far stronger instrument in God's service.

Every soul disease is then an aggregation of thoughts which together create a form. The form of the soul disease can be recognized in the soul's different vehicles, as the symptoms become manifest through the vital force's work to preserve the economy of the vehicles. The form of the soul disease has the ability to affect the form (to change it) of the vehicles, as witnessed clearly in the grossest soul manifestation, the physical vehicle.

It follows, then, that any disease manifesting in the physical, emotional, or mental bodies, even when pathology exists (meaning now there are not only functional changes but structural changes also), can be reversed and health can be attained, if and only if the soul disease is healed through consciousness. The soul disease was created by lack of consciousness, therefore only consciousness (a shattering of ego delusion and desires and a return to one's divine connection) can bring about a healing.

Microscopes and advanced technology will aid us to see the disease results, even the finest, such as bacteria and viruses, the finest forms of animal or vegetable life, but they will always only help us to see the physical (or mental/emotional) manifest outcome of disease. They cannot illuminate us as to the real disease origin, which is seated in the soul.

Bacteria are beneficent agents in the Cosmos. If the terrain is dirty, the bacteria will proliferate. This does not only refer to the fluids of the body – the blood and lymph etc., but also to the emotional, mental and spiritual terrain. Bacteria exist as positive constructive agents. If there is a weakening of one of the soul's vehicles, due to a lack of consciousness and therefore an inverted lifestyle, poor eating and thinking habits etc., there will be a susceptibility in the individual and the bacteria will find ground to establish themselves and propagate and will execute their usual "clean-up recycling" act instead of in a dead body, in a live one, thus degenerative processes are set in action.

Read Robert Young's book, *Sick and Tired.* Bacteria have a pleomorphic ability. They assume forms, shapes and functions according to the environment. They can become constructive red blood cells which can be transformed into any cell needed by the body in a healthy positive environment, or they can become yeast, fungus, mold and eventually be the cause of the death of the body. When they destroy a body, they are merely performing their task of recycling excessive waste, even though the body still happens to have life. The bacteria operate under the same fixed energetic Cosmic Laws as man.

Susceptibility

The true cause of disease is a lack of consciousness. All the bodies are so intrinsically connected that whatever is experienced in the mental and emotional realms, is reflected to a greater or lesser degree in the physical realm, depending on the strength of the physical body.

Susceptibility is the reaction of the organism to external and internal influence. If there is any weakness in a person, susceptibility exists in the area of weakness. **You attract what you need in order for you to grow strong.** You suffer owing to what you attract because you attract that which is most difficult for you to overcome i.e. your weakness. The same stimulus does not affect others exposed to it as they are not susceptible to it (there is no weakness). Balance of all the bodies, which is strength, will always be the greatest protection. The negative energy, which must be regarded as a strengthening energy necessary to evolution, will always assail us at an opportune moment, impelling us to overcome the adversity and so evolve. You get strong if you overpower the morbidity you attracted, or weaker if it overpowers you. Any adversity that you are successful in surpassing, will strengthen you, bestowing you with a greater immunity to like adversity in the future, be it bacterial or an emotional stress such as grief or disappointment. On the physical level, the bacteria can only affect you i.e. flourish and proliferate if your inner terrain is unbalanced (too acidic, electromagnetically weak, etc.) On the emotional level, the stress can only affect you if you are emotionally weak i.e. lacking in spiritual vision.

For instance, if a girl is subjected to mild sexual abuse but she is too timid to speak up at the time or perhaps part of her even enjoys it and therefore does not put an end to it or speak about it afterwards. She projects her feelings of anger towards the offender and harbors guilt feelings herself, but the incident remains hidden and unresolved. The situation overpowered her, she did not have the strength to overcome it, for whatever reason, but she now has fear perhaps coupled with guilt and will most likely attract the same or a similar situation again. She is therefore still susceptible to this particular adversity so must live the experience in order to get strong, although the experience could come in a completely different form the next time. When we have strengthened ourselves sufficiently by succeeding in overcoming the adversities we are given, we are no longer susceptible to those adversities. However, perhaps we are exposed to the same adversity but in a higher intensity. At this intensity we are still susceptible and overcome, but we will have the tools to fight and ward it off this time; we are a lot stronger. This applies equally to physical, emotional and mental morbific stimuli.

In the perfect Divine Plan, we are never confronted with negativity which is impossible for us to overcome. There is always a Universal Justice at play, although from our limited perspective (our imperfect mind-filtered vision, in addition to our vision which only expands the length of one life time on one dimension), this may not appear to be true. A good example would be a person who is plagued by unresolved resentment and anger towards her father, which extends to her husband in the course of her marriage, and this together with incorrect eating habits centered around comfort eating rather than healthy diet, results in a slow insidious cancer development, which after many years threatens to destroy her life. The person is forced to decide between the diverse allopathic and alternative treatments and after much consideration, opts for naturopathy and homeopathy. She learns how to eat right, natural therapies to cleanse her body, learns to forgive and release the negative emotions, is helped with energy cures or homeopathic remedies and her consciousness expands. However, she sought treatment too late and her vital force is not strong enough to fight the necrotic cancer that has invaded and corroded her body. She dies. We would conclude that she was defeated because she was overwhelmed by a negative force too powerful for her to combat. But seeing this woman's Earth life as but one fragment of her evolution, we would be able to view the situation entirely differently. She passed on to another dimension with a different consciousness, with a different will, with different life and thought habits and patterns. She will return to Earth to complete her chakra life lessons, a stronger more conscious person; she is already a transformed more conscious person.

It is not so much what happens to us but how we confront the situation. Our attitude is what is important. We may die and all of humanity may think that we failed, but actually we died in triumph or we may live by devious means and apparently we are victorious but actually our acts were self-defeating in evolutionary terms. We have to have the eye of the spirit, not Earth programming, in our assessments.

Never forget the energetic law: we attract what we need for our well-being, however we do not always recognize the fact that what we have attracted may cause us pain in our endeavors to overcome it, even though it serves our growth and well-being. No leaf falls to the ground without it being part of the cosmic order – there are no co-incidences; there is no good or bad luck. We are all interconnected and within this intimate interconnection, we all receive what we require, when we require it, synchronistically, for our evolution.

Free will always exists, so we can choose to fall into a degenerate lifestyle because of disappointments and sorrows; not everyone is evolving (meaning ascending vibrationally) all the time. Energy is never stationary; we are either evolving or devolving. Ascension is not easy but it is deeply fulfilling and rewarding. Involution cannot be easy either; it is fraught with pain and suffering. When you are working hard in your ascension, you feel the perfection of creation, you feel one with it, even though you are aware that what you are doing is not easy, you feel that anything asked of you from above is possible, if you love and care

17

enough, if you yearn to serve humanity in the way that God has asked you to.

Delusions

The ego is what stands between you and God. The ego is meant to be constructed in Chakras 1, 2 and 3 and then shattered in Chakras 4, 5 and 6. A perfect balance is meant to be attained in Ch. 7. Few people have balanced egos, most have superiority or inferiority complexes. Many people compensate feelings of inferiority by manifesting with inflated egos and many of these people even land up believing their own acts.

In the aftermath of the devastating negative era which went evil, many people have lost their hearts, their love energy. To understand and help another person, you have to see life through his consciousness so that you really feel and understand the person. You cannot just put yourself, with your consciousness, in his shoes. You have to don his shoes in order to understand him.

Love is life. There is no life without love. There is survival and existence but not life. Love is the magical transformative energy of life. In order to guide a person to his healing, you have to enter his shoes and consciousness, and then love him.

Love is union, it is the fabric of real life. Separation and segregation are pain. Egos separate, isolate and segregate. A balanced ego is positive and necessary. Unbalanced egos have caused all the pain in the Cosmos. Egos create blindness which creates delusions and then these same delusions are self-perpetuated by the egos. There is no healing without recognizing the delusion and shattering it.

Common delusions:

Delusion: Love is weakness; power is strength. Acts of love and giving are viewed as a weakness whereas the exercise of power and the demanding of respect through fear, is seen as strength.

Truth: Respect is earned and only one who possesses love will be able to govern with justice, without instilling fear.

Delusion: I have to cover up my weaknesses or I will not be loved and accepted, I will be rejected. I have to uphold my image of strength.

Truth: Egos are not lovable; transparency is comprehendible and therefore lovable. Being transparent is a strength not a weakness. Masking your insecurities and anxieties with a façade of self-confidence, makes you unloving and unlovable. Your energy is so consumed in maintaining your mask, your posture of strength, that you are unable to feel and therefore love others. All your energies are self-directed, weakening you.

Delusion (Of contrived or inhibited people who find it so difficult to be natural, to be themselves): Others are scrutinizing, judging and criticizing me. Thoughts when with others: How am I coming across? What are they thinking of me right now? Can they tell how weird or uncomfortable I feel? I'm sure they can, etc.

Truth: You scrutinize, judge and criticize others all the time and you project those feelings onto them, believing that everyone is like that. Most people are not even noticing or thinking about you at all, they are busy with their own lives. If you would stop criticizing others mentally, you would liberate yourself of all inhibitions. If you speak your mind and are open and direct with others, questioning whatever you do not understand or perhaps agree with, you would not harbor negative thoughts in the first place, they would be spoken and would not be negative and charged, they would be questions. These projections are common e.g. someone who is sex obsessed thinks that others are too and misconstrues their words or gestures, believing them to have sexual connotations.

Delusion: I am a bad person. Or I am a good person.

Truth: There are no absolutely good or bad people; we all have the potential to become either energy predominantly, as we all possess the duality. However, there are good and bad actions. The most balanced person (a balanced Ch. 7 person) is one who is closest to a 50-50 ratio of Cosmic Energy (the commitment, love energy) and Kundalini Energy (the discipline energy of strength). Such a balanced person would be able to understand, identify and therefore respond appropriately to both energies.

Delusion: I am really special. God favors me. He loves me more than others.

Truth: God loves everyone equally but helps those who help Him to help others more, out of necessity, because He loves all of humanity and wants them helped. He is only able to guide (help) those who are open to his guidance and who obey it. He is also only able to help those who have learned how to connect and therefore hear his guidance well.

Delusion: I am extremely smart. I am very talented. I am highly knowledgeable, capable, etc.

Truth: The Cosmos is so vast. The smaller our minds, the greater our tunnel vision, the more self-centered our energies, the bigger the ego and the more self-deluded and blind we are. The more our energies are centrifugally directed (outwards towards others), the more aware we are, the more easily we connect to others on this and higher dimensions, the more impossible it becomes to have these delusions, even if we are talented in certain areas. Most people are talented in specific areas, depending on what we have focused on most in life. We will know our strong areas and our weak areas but we will know many others who are stronger than ourselves even in our strong areas. We will realize the infinite number of areas we have never even tackled. The bigger the mind, the higher the consciousness, the more impossible it is to have a big ego.

Delusion: I am so spiritual. I wake up at 5 a.m. daily, do Pranayama, Hatha Yoga, then Meditations. I dedicate my life to selfless service. I eat a light, healthy diet, etc.

Truth: Maybe you are and maybe you are not. Your connection to your own Higher Self, your guide, God, Jesus, Buddha or whoever you feel closest to, will determine how spiritual you really are. Your spirituality can be gauged by the measure in which you are guided from a more evolved being from a higher dimension, and follow the guidance, which will always lead you to your ascension. The closer you approximate Ch. 6, the spirit, the farther you are from Ch. 1, money or matter, the more spiritual you are. In Chakra 7 you are able to attain a high spiritual level, living in balance with the material personal chakras 1, 2 and 3. The easier a person is able to connect and communicate with others deeply; the more s/he can perceive and feel others, the more his/her reactions and responses to others are appropriate, the more spiritual s/he is. The more a person loves others before himself, the less ego he has, the more spiritual he is.

Delusion: I have a loose wire. I cannot concentrate. I have never liked mental work, I find it so difficult to comprehend and remember information I read. This can be applied to any area in life. I am the worst cook and I never even remember to eat, I'm always too busy. I hate the kitchen and find it such a waste of time. I hate meditating. It's such a waste of time. I need to get through my to do list of the day rather.

Truth: Any resistance reflects an area that has never been worked much, therefore never mastered, and therefore is not enjoyed. We enjoy things that come easily to us, so we enjoy the areas we have worked in past lives or in this life. Most people avoid the same chakra life lessons lifetime after lifetime and overdo the ones they are energetically attuned to. We need to be patient with our resistance areas and work them daily, little by little, not avoid them, and after a certain amount of time we will be surprised at how we develop a passion and love for them. Most people on Earth are weak in the love, commitment, dedication, devotion, surrender energy chakras – 2, 4 and 6. I surrender my will to Thy will, Father. I unite my will to Thine. I surrender personal desires and live in Thy service for Thy Divine Plan.

Delusion: I am weak thanks to my far from ideal childhood. My parents were unbalanced and they inculcated the wrong beliefs and habits in me from young.

Truth: You earned your parents according to your level of consciousness. You also chose them because of the lessons you needed to learn in order to overcome, strengthening you. Nothing is chance. There are no victims in life. The justice of the Divine Plan never fails. We are never dealt life lessons that are too difficult for us to cope with.

Delusion: Physical appearance is extremely important. I must spend the rest of my life with someone truly beautiful/ handsome. I admire and respect beautiful people over plain or ugly people and everyone does.

Truth: Beauty is in the eyes of the beholder. This will always stand true. When you love someone deeply, that person becomes physically beautiful to you. If you do not, even the most perfect person physically, will not seem beautiful to you after some time. You will always find more beautiful people than yourself, partner or children (also less beautiful). On Earth, the more kundalini energy you have, the more attuned you are to the negative energy on Earth, the better you will fare physically. In the cosmic world, one's appearance is more related to one's love and strength energies. Aging is not known in the light worlds. The more positive the world, meaning the higher its positive standards, and the stronger the person, meaning the more positive they are, the less the person will age. Aging and death of plants, animals and man only occurs in negative worlds, due to the negative energy. On Earth, the most loving and therefore happiest people, are those who are able to easily see and feel the inner beauty in others.

It is only possible to be in love with someone whose consciousness is at your level, or higher. To be in love with someone, you must respect and admire the person. We can love many people but we can only feel deeply in love with a man or woman who possesses a level of consciousness we deeply admire. The physical can and does change on any dimension. One's consciousness is what is enduring.

Delusion: I just have to finish . . . and then I'll enter spiritual life.

Truth: The list is never ending. You'll finish one thing and want to finish the next and never enter your spiritual life unless you realize this.

Delusion: I am intuitive. I'm guided in my life, etc.

Truth: Many people are intuitive to varying degrees but you are not guided in your life unless you have learnt to receive very detailed specific instructions from an evolved being on a higher dimension. You may have learnt to receive the instructions and still not be guided. You have to receive the guidance twice a day and follow it and then you know you are leading a guided life.

Delusion: My mission in life is to travel and connect people to each other. This can be applied to any life situation – e.g. my mission in life is to have a family. My mission in life is to travel the world performing energy cures and visiting the important energy zones on the planet. My mission in life is to be a spiritual teacher (and the children are neglected for the important mission) etc.

Truth: Everyone's first and foremost mission is to learn to connect so we receive our guidance and mission. Once we are connected and receiving guidance minimum twice a day, we will be guided as to exactly what to do with our lives. Know that your guidance is correct if it always guides you to your own purification and strengthening and to service to others. It demands self-discipline and will only be of benefit to you and your loved ones, ascending you all.

"Delusions – It is only highly egotistical and ego mania people who can develop delusions and this is the reason: a person who is so intolerant of the views of other people, who always believes he is right, that he knows best, cannot accept any new ideas, is not even receptive to them, even though they may be correct and beneficial. This leads to a state of mind which excludes the possibility of seeing the truth. In such an instance, the qualities of clarity and creative service are lacking and are preventing the full and proper use of his mental faculties. Progressively, such a person is prone to develop a state of delusion, a state in which the false appears to him to be true. In this way, the highly egotistical and selfish person paves the way for a state of confusion which may eventually lead to a state of actual insanity.

We can see a similar process in a highly acquisitive individual. This person has great belief in material value; nothing is more important than the possessions he desires to acquire – which may be objects or people. Such possessiveness may evolve into a driving desire so out of proportion to reality that the person may seek satisfaction at any cost. Exploitation of others, or even harm to others, will not be sufficient obstacles once the desire becomes obsessive. A person in this state has lost all idealistic and ethical values." (George Vithoulkas, *The Science of Homeopathy.*)

Deep-seated delusional beliefs keep people negative and incurable. Everyone thinks of sickness as all the chronic and degenerative physical diseases because everyone only sees and feels the physical, they don't have the eyes or feel capacity to see and feel all the deeply sick emotional, mental and spiritual body cases. These are the deeply sick cases because they are never helped, as they never look for help. The greater the chaos, the less efficient the person, the less the inner harmony, the greater the awkwardness and inhibitions, the less the feel capacity, the greater the weakness and negativity. Not all these factors have to be present but they are good indicators of emotionally or mentally sick people.

The best indicator of emotional and mental health is naturalness and spontaneity of expression, warmth and freedom of expression. The more bound the person, the greater the mask, the less they can feel others because the more they are so in themselves. Anyone with a mask, is only masking negativity. The thicker the mask, the greater the negativity being masked. There are different forms of unnatural, different masks, but they all hide (mask) negativity.

Emotional Body Healing

One cleanses and strengthens through correct life disciplines (see Cosmic Reawakening) and by getting out of yourself and giving to others. Cleansing consist of opening up and expressing all the accumulated and often highly embarrassing garbage. The three steps in order of depth are: written, verbal with eyes closed, and verbal with eyes open. The deeper the cleanse, the more your life disciplines will be able to move and ascend you and the more you will be able to give to others, because the more you will begin to recuperate your feel capacity.

You have to be constantly cleansing and strengthening. This requires living in consciousness (so stop talking as much as is possible). The more you strengthen after a cleanse, meaning the more conscientious you are with your disciplines, the deeper your next cleanse will be.

In theory it's very simple — as something surfaces that you feel remorseful about, cleanse it. Strengthen through disciplines so that you are constantly changing yourself. Disciplines include mental disciplines such as eliminating negative destructive thoughts. As you strengthen and change yourself, your consciousness will expand and you'll be conscious of more incidents that you are remorseful about. Cleanse again.

You should not apologize (cleanse) unless you are sure that you will not repeat that same mistake. Strengthening also entails acquiring the necessary skills that you need in order to stop repeating the same errors (parenting, teaching, opening and connecting to people, etc.) There are cycles of greater cleansing and those of more strengthening, but the two processes should really be occurring simultaneously too throughout your life.

These are the transformative emotional body steps that we found successful in Tashirat:

1. Confessions about your Earth life and get in touch with your Cosmic life past too, if possible. Recognize patterns and confront who you really are and what your motivations in life have been.

2. Verbally expose and apologize.

3. If the person cannot apologize sincerely, then she must come up with all the justifications that prevent her from feeling remorse for whatever has been done and then work to knock the justifications.

4. If the person is so lacking in feeling, then he must find whatever he is sorry for (regardless of how significant or insignificant the things may seem). All feelings of remorse must be exposed so that he can start feeling and exposing more – i.e. cleansing.

5. The person must expose her negative thoughts all the time and write the correct arguments, knocking the thoughts. If the same thoughts keep repeating, then the person does not have the conviction of her arguments.

6. Fight the negative thoughts or voices out loud. Come up with proper strong arguments and fight back with conviction. Continue with written arguments daily.

7. For pride – the person must expose everything that he is proud of about himself or his accomplishments. If he thinks that he is so great, he must expose and explain why to everyone, who will then try and show him how illogical his delusional beliefs are. He has to also expose all of his deepest desires and beliefs.

8. Now the person has seen himself unmasked. He must learn to be real in life and never again fall into the habit of wearing a mask.

THE PROCESS OF GETTING REAL

a. The person is given a reference point of who they really are. They are provoked so that their mask is broken and they are able to see who they really are.
b. It is easy for people to criticize others, so they are encouraged to, in order to become real.
c. Once the person is real, she must expose herself from her real unmasked self. She must compare herself to others and expose everything that she feels ashamed about, that she doesn't want anyone to know. She must expose her likes, dislikes and delusions.
d. The delusions can only be broken from the real unmasked place, from the negative real person. Every delusion has to be broken mentally first but then through the exposure job it should get broken at a gut level.
e. To stay real in life, the person must have the courage to always express his truth. From the real you, you say what you want to change and why and start changing.

Vanity as the Root of all Evil

The belief system that stems from all negative worlds, is that model beauty is power and people only love, respect and admire beautiful people. Sadly enough, this is true in negative worlds, such as the Earth. Negative worlds uphold values such as appearance, power and sensual living, and because of it, these people have lost the ability to feel and to love. They cannot penetrate and feel the essence beauty in people, which is what really makes people appear beautiful. As negative world people are so physically-anchored, and have no emotional or spiritual bodies, they can and do only go by physical appearance.

There are few model looking people and those who are, are too frequently some of the sickest, saddest people. There are few really gorgeous people who are truly unassuming and spiritual. People with negative world values often lack self-confidence, even when they are good-looking, because there are always better looking people, wherever you go. They are excruciatingly self-critical about their own physical appearance and envious of the beauty others possess. They never feel perfect enough physically. So much of their time and energy is consumed, as they are weakened in their evolution, by their physical beauty obsession.

Some of the greatest people on Earth, the most loved, respected and admired people, were no models. Abraham Lincoln was one of the most physically unattractive men. No women looked at him until his wife had the eyes to see beyond his looks. Mother Theresa, who cared for the poor she served, cared only to serve God through her noble work. Do you think she would have chosen model beauty nuns to help her in her service or wholesome nuns with a heart? She embraced positive world values and that's why her and her nuns wore the robe and head-dress they chose to wear, so as not to focus on the physical. She and Gandhi were happy, fulfilled people who truly contributed to this world. Einstein went to public lectures with his disheveled hair and in slippers. His mind was elsewhere.

When people from the light cosmic world go on missions and work on negative planets (like Earth or on the second dimension), their appearance soon changes. The lighter and more positive they are, the faster their physical appearance deteriorates in a negative energy environment. However, when they return, if they returned from a mission on their dimension, so didn't lose their body, their physical transforms again and they are even more beautiful than before because of their newly acquired strength and purity, thanks to their experience. Appearances in light worlds change according to your soul qualities.

How one sees is all a matter of consciousness. One's vision reflects who one is, it reflects one's consciousness. People who only love and admire physical beauty and criticize all else, are miserable people. People who are only happy with themselves when they feel physically perfect, are deeply unhappy people. The root of bulimia and anorexia is vanity. These highly critical, judgmental people have never known love and cannot until they change deeply, radically, from within. Women are more prone to vanity than men. As soon as you start feeling people, your vision changes, and a whole world of true beauty opens to you.

The root of all evil is not necessarily money, I believe it's vanity. Pride and vanity have committed horrendous war crimes, creating so much unnecessary suffering. Vanity is related to so many of the evils of Chakras 1 and 2. Vanity is one of the main roots of a loveless, mindless, unhappy life. In negative worlds, vanity reigns. If you want to live a positive, happy life, steer clear of the dangers of vanity. Vain people are twisted, lonely souls who do not find the happiness they are seeking, because happiness is only found in love. This is universal.

Looking for happiness in power, recognition, beauty, possessions, sensual pleasures, etc. will only result in ultimate disappointment. Only pure love, knowledge and deep spirituality will ever fill the void that people who lack this, feel. When you know how to love and you really love someone, that person is beautiful to you. Even if the person has physical or emotional body defects, if you are in love with him/her, you will even love the defects.

If your value system, your heart and mind, are full of love and true beauty; if you attain health of the physical AND other bodies, you will shine not with a model perfect features body and face but with a God-radiance of a balanced human being full of knowledge, love and inner plenitude. You will feel full of self-confidence and will be content with your appearance and not envy others better physically looking than yourself.

In the end, we each live our soul/heart/mind deep desires and attract to ourselves people and experiences of our vibration. This is the Cosmic Justice than never errs.

The Law of Attraction

What you think about most, you will attract and become. You will either attract your worst fears or your greatest desires. Whatever is happening in your mind, you are attracting. Your thoughts formulate your future experience. Thoughts are frequencies and if consistently repeated, they become things. If you emit that frequency consistently, you will attract it. You attract the predominant thought you hold in your mind.

A positive thought is far more powerful than a negative thought. Don't monitor your thoughts, there are too many. Monitor your emotions. If you feel good and happy, then what you are thinking is in line with what you want. It is a good frequency. And the converse. You can know how in alignment you are by how you feel. It is easier to know what you are feeling about rather than what you are thinking about. *What you think, what you feel, and what manifests, will always match. Whatever you can conceive, you can achieve.*

Whatever you really want, you will receive. Any fantasy can be turned into a fact. The how and when you leave to the universe. Just know that you'll acquire or achieve whatever you want depending on how badly you want it and how single-minded you are in your desire. It helps to visualize because when you visualize, you materialize. If you go there in the mind, you'll go there in the body. Focus on your dream, allow it to consume you, to guide and sustain you. Feed it constantly by thinking about it and having it in mind always. Your dream must be the driving force behind all you do. It is all feeling, not so much thinking. Feel your dream.

Always only dwell upon the end result. It's the feeling that creates the attraction. Feel the joy and happiness when accomplishing your dream. The power of the universe can enter and express when you see and feel well enough. Feel exhilarated by the whole creative process. Be consistent with feeling high, exhilarated and happy, knowing that you will definitely accomplish your dream. Visualize it and know that it is already acquired.

You should be living with a sense of inner joy, peace, happiness and the rest will naturally happen. Your primary aim in life is to experience joy, freedom, love, happiness, laughter. Do what gives you all of this constantly. Inner happiness is the fuel for success. Anything that makes you feel good and happy, is attracting more goodness and happiness into your life.

Our body is a reflection of our thoughts and emotions. All disease (dis-ease, dis-harmony) is due to stress. Believe it in your heart and follow the natural laws of healing, and you will be healed. Avoid all stress. Laugh a lot. Disease cannot survive in a person with a healthy emotional state. See yourself living in a perfectly healthy body. Stress and negative thoughts degrade the body. Positive thoughts reconstruct the body. Have the belief that you are getting younger, not older. Be aware of your own infinite nature. Live from your heart and go for what you want in life. Convert your want into your reality. Don't focus on what you don't want, only on what you do want. Have the firm belief that everything always goes right for you and all is well in the Cosmos.

Whether you think you can or can't, either way you are right (Henry Ford). Live in a different reality. With the Law of Attraction nothing is impossible. Follow your bliss (Joseph Campbell).

Chakras

Strength and Balance Numbers

CHAKRA 1

Strength – The ability to make money. The passion and intensity with which you love your work.

Balance – How you utilize and administrate it i.e. how organized you are and whether it is employed for the good of others (humanity) or yourself (your family).

CHAKRA 2

EMOTIONAL

Strength – The intensity of your love for your husband/wife. How submissive or domineering you are with your partner.

Balance - How loving, giving, caring you are. How physically affectionate you are. How aware you are emotionally of your partner. How well you are able to fulfill his/her emotional needs. How sensitive, perceptive and emotionally switched on consistently you are with your partner. As a male, this will also depend on you possessing predominantly the strong protective KE, but having sufficient loving, sensitive, giving CE. As a female, it will depend on you having a strong soft, loving, perceptive, intuitive CE, but having sufficient strong KE, so that you have your own life interests and opinions, and are not an overly submissive wife that the husband cannot respect.

PHYSICAL

Strength – Entirely dependent on the physical strength of Ch. 3.

Balance – How considerate you are with your partner sexually. How much you give and how much you demand. How sensitive you are to your partner's physical needs and how well you fulfill them (or selfishly fulfill your own needs more).

CHAKRA 3

PHYSICAL

Strength – Dependent on correct nutrition and exercise. A healthy balanced personalized diet, correct for the individual's vibration, evolution and predominant current chakra life lesson. Sufficient exercise corresponding to the person's physical health, vibration, evolution and predominant current chakra life lesson. The lower the person's vibration, the more the biochemical aspect of food is important. The higher the vibration, the more the vibrational aspect of food is significant.

Balance – Whether you undereat, overeat or are moderate in your eating habits, eating healthily to nourish the body. Whether you do not exercise enough daily, or exercise in excess or are moderate in your daily exercise regime. Your motives are highly indicative of balance or imbalance. Overexercising and undereating because of vanity. Under exercising and eating anything the moment you are starving because your focus in life is excessively mental and the physical is neglected.

EMOTIONAL

Strength – How emotionally balanced and competent you are as a person and therefore as a parent. The intensity of your love for your children. You are meant to be all giving, this is your role, and expect nothing more than love, respect and admiration from your children, all of which had to have been earned, never demanded, by being the person you are. Your children will know you by your living example, not by your lengthy lectures and will follow your example more than your words. Your emotional strength will depend on your level of sensitivity, perception, intuition and ability to love. It will also depend on your expertise regarding health and hygiene. Your knowledge of Naturopathy and ability to keep yourself and your family healthy.

Balance - How dominant/submissive (strict/liberal) you are and how sensitive you are to your own and therefore your child's emotional needs regarding diet.

CHAKRA 4

Strength – Your desire to help humanity. Your love and service to people other than your immediate family or personal friends. How easily you make the Chakra 4 jump, because of your desire to help humanity. Your attachment to lower chakras (family in particular) will affect your Chakra 4 strength. The intensity of your love for your spiritual team.

Balance – How much you give to your spiritual team happily, with love and no ego, fulfilling any task needed by the team. Do you over-give, under-give or are you balanced in your giving and service? How much you embrace your spiritual team as your family.

CHAKRA 5

Strength – Your mental capacity. The greater your global vision, the greater will be your mental clarity and ability to transmit this clarity. It will determine your ability to extract the essence from a wealth of information read and organize it into a coherent clearly comprehensible whole. Your desire to impart the knowledge to others and the intensity of your love for your students.

Balance – The ability to transmit knowledge in a creative, interesting, concise, clear manner. The ability to teach, which will depend on the strength and balance of your emotional and mental bodies and whether you are too dominant or submissive as a teacher (meaning as a person).

CHAKRA 6

Strength – The intensity of your love for humanity and God. The degree of surrendering your will and uniting it to God's. Your degree of connection – hearing by feeling and knowing the truth of what you hear by being able to identify the energy accompanying what you hear.

Balance – Whether you are too dedicated, submissive, giving and obedient to God (or your Higher Self or any teacher of advanced evolution on a higher dimension or your spiritual teacher on this dimension), blindly following the guidance given or whether you are not submissive enough, doing your own thing, not asking enough questions because you really want to do your own thing. Not surrendering your will enough to the Divine Will. Not being able to relinquish your personal desires, meaning still having too much ego to really be spiritual.

CHAKRA 7

Strength – Will depend on the strength of all the other chakras.

Balance – Will depend on the strength and balance of all the other chakras.

One is meant to surrender one's will, to unite one's will to God's in Chakras 1 to 6. Do not exert your will at all, surrender your desires and unite your will fully to God's. Of course to do this, you have to be able to hear His will, hence the necessity of learning to connect. In Chakra 7 you must balance what you receive from God with what you think is correct for your living experience. In other words, only in Chakra 7, do you learn to balance your will and what you think and believe, with God's will, with His guidance. However, even in Chakra 7, beware of exerting your will too much. Rather discuss your thoughts with Him and listen to His arguments really carefully before making a final decision.

Ascension

A cure takes place when a person's vibration is raised. There is no panacea diet, treatment or lifestyle. Everything depends on the individual's energy, past history, present condition and habits etc. So many factors are involved. Therefore each treatment has to be highly individualized and ideally the person guiding the treatment must be connected and have access to the person's cosmic past.

However, what is universal, is that a cure is achieved, when whatever the treatment, it raises the person's vibration slightly above his current vibration. For any permanent cure to take place, self-discipline and therefore an expanded consciousness, is necessary. The higher a person's consciousness from a past life, the more will be required to achieve a successful healing. A person who did not attain Ch. 4 and above in a past life, could easily be healed from an advanced cancer by only following dietary and natural therapy instructions, with some emotional changes. This would not be the case for a cancer patient who has achieved a Ch. 4 or above consciousness in a past life. This chapter deals with ascension for patients or spiritual aspirants. Many patients become spiritual aspirants and are obviously healed in their ascension journey. For any patient to be healed, ascension is essential.

Life is never simply easy if you are ascending. Unless you are descending, and most people are through their lifetimes, although slowly, don't expect the going to be easy. The majority take the easy route of least resistance – they do what they are good at, avoid what they cannot master and are not focusing on evolving. And even the easy route is fraught with disappointment, disillusion and pain, so it isn't really so easy, it's difficult actually and you are surrounded by people who are mostly impure and/or weak.

Ascension is not easy, it entails confronting every single weak area of yours – every weak chakra life lesson. The area first has to be cleansed, which for some people takes years. And once cleansed, it must be strengthened. So no-one can expect the path of ascension to be easy. Along the way, there are little hurdles to jump and big seemingly insurmountable blockades that have to be overcome and then there are some smooth periods, always after jumping a mound, but all the while you are ascending, never descending the mountain and if you do descend at all, you just have to climb up again and do double work. When you do manage to scale a difficult ridge or you discover a way of climbing a steep and torturous ascending path, you feel accomplished and elated because your panoramic view is so amplified, so extended, and you comprehend so much more and from now on you will live at a higher level of peace and happiness. But if you are on the speedy path of evolution, this cosmic path, and you are only focusing on ascending, not at stopping and admiring or studying the landscape or vegetation or anything else, although you do this too as you are ascending, then you are sure to confront another obstacle soon. All obstacles really are but a test of your ingenuity and strength. They come in different sizes and forms – thorny bushes seemingly impossible to traverse, inclines too steep to climb, foliage thick and abounding in insects, etc. But there is no obstacle that cannot be overcome, you just have to find the best way to overcome it. Sometimes past experience helps, other times a whole new approach is required.

If you love God and only want to unite your will to His and only want to purify and strengthen yourself so you are able to serve Him well, then you will never doubt your tough ascension. You will never get angry at the obstacles, you will never feel deprived of the pleasures others who have not chosen to ascend God's evolutionary mountain appear to be living, you will never for one moment forget what you are doing and you will also never expect climbing the mountain to be easy and always joyful or pleasurable, although there will be times of the greatest joy and happiness, times of real ecstasy. Whilst up against a crunch, life won't be joyful but as soon as you are through the crisis, you will be filled with gratitude for this Mountain of Evolution that was constructed to fortify you.

Each obstacle encountered, whether it requires looking deeply and honestly at yourself and cleansing, or whether it requires strengthening, can be overcome. There never was or will be an insurmountable obstacle because there are many ways to overcome every obstacle, you just have to find the way that best suits you. But it definitely can and must be overcome. Ascension will always be fraught with obstacles – they are your evolutionary tests. So few people are prepared to keep ascending. Most climb for a time and then surrender and hope to hold on to the consciousness of the view they attained, as they descend and go and live at the bottom of the mountain with the masses. Sadly, it doesn't work like this. You lose the view and vision you attained rapidly, as you descend.

You can live with God, serving Him, working with and for Him, at the top of the mountain, but you have to be willing to pay the price, and for such a great life, you have to keep ascending until Ch. 7 has been completed and then you are home and God can use you for His work, and your mission on Earth begins. To keep ascending without surrender, requires considerable stamina, exceptional certainty of purpose, consistent perseverance, keeping your goal ever present in mind, and forever working hard.

Climbing the evolutionary mountain requires great physical endurance, emotional stability, tremendous love for God and the Divine Cosmic Plan and its Creator, and inordinate mental ability. Those who determine to climb and keep climbing are the free spirits who actually one day attain liberation from all enslaving chains, who follow only their desire to serve God and the Divine Plan. They are the ones who succeed. Never expect the ascension to be easy, for if it were, everyone would be ascending. It's a mammoth task which requires exceptional dexterity of every body , and yes there is sufferance along the way for all hikers. However, if you keep the goal in mind, there will always be a sense of deep fulfillment, as you know where you are going in life and why. And whilst ascending, you are meant to be in close communication with God or your spiritual guide or whoever you are close to from a higher level, and they are meant to be assisting you every step of the way, because everyone knows, ascension is not an easy task. But for every step you actually ascend, there is no losing it unless you lose hope one day and decide to surrender and you slide down the mountain "happily," relieved that you no longer have to exert yourself to that extent ever again in your life. And life becomes a blur of activities. However, your focus is no longer ascension and so you are not ascending at the pace you were when you were aware that you were climbing and you felt the demanding exertion. In this "happy" life, you are fortunate if you do ascend at all. Most people descend and get weaker each lifetime, as the negative pull of the worldly attractions is too great.

It is so much easier to ascend with other climbers who are also ascending. Although it is difficult for everyone and no-one is living a pleasurable joy ride, at least they are all climbing and going up, so neither the path nor the mountain climbers are luring you downhill.

Each one's obstacles are different, but anyone who has sufficient determination, will look beyond the obstacle, even when in the thick of an apparently insurmountable one, and never lose hope. "if I do my utmost, really my utmost, I know by energetic law, I will be helped over this obstacle too," must always be your attitude. But how much are you prepared to give before getting angry, before surrendering? You have to keep giving your all until God deems it the correct moment to help you.

He cannot and will not help you one second before you have given your all, because He would be violating the Laws, depriving you of your force.

So this evolutionary journey is not for everyone. It is not for the fainthearted. It is not for victims. It is not for those who aren't prepared to fight and work arduously, for those who are mad at whoever or whatever circumstance in life. Each person in your life, each circumstance, is an opportunity to look deeper and with greater acuity at yourself, because while ascending the weaknesses in each body will become blatantly apparent. What was not that apparent on the flat plane life at the bottom of the mountain, is now magnified many times, as your every muscle, every sense is taut with the overexertion of your relentless ascent. It is for each one to decide whether s/he possesses the caliber of an evolutionary mountain climber.

Never endeavor to climb without props. God and your guide are your props. No-one can ascend alone. Through the fog, through the storms, the thorns and jagged rocks, you have to find a way, even when at your worst, to hear God or your guide and follow the guidance, because it's when the going gets tough that it's most difficult to hear. However, you can and have to. Before trying to hear, remember your purpose in life, which is the only thing in the confusion which will lift the fog and black clouds, and balance you, thereby enabling you to be guided.

Even when the path is impossibly difficult and you cannot see your way out, just keep plodding, exert to maximum capacity, don't expect help, know that you have to make the supreme effort, but if you keep going long enough, there is no doubt, you will be helped if and when help is needed. That is what strength is. That is what faith is. No-one made it to the pinnacle without either strength or faith. Both ingredients are required. Accept every obstacle, every challenge that presents itself, without anger or despair. Accept it and keep walking, keeping working to find a way through it. That is what evolution is all about. Don't demand help from God or anyone, with love and humility ask God or anyone else for guidance. No person or circumstance ever weakened you. You are not a victim. You allowed yourself to be weakened. Now it's up to you to work hard to strengthen yourself. Ignorance is not a valid justification. We pay a high penalty for ignorance, we learn the hard way, through sufferance. Live to learn and dispel ignorance.

Become a steadfast, stalwart Warrior of Light. Prove yourself by becoming an unwavering, stable mountain climber. With each triumph, your ascension does not become easier, as ascension is never easy, but your inner fire and steel augment and there is less chance of you becoming despondent enough to slide down. The higher you ascend, the less likely you are to become fainthearted for too long, as your comprehension is greater, as is your determination to succeed.

Regarding marijuana, peyote and other drugs: on the Cosmic Path we believe in using our own force to raise our vibration – in purifying and strengthening enough to ascend, thus being able to receive guidance from our own Higher Self, our spiritual guide, God, Jesus or any other evolved soul we feel in tune with. We do not believe in seeking psychic experiences, on the contrary, we believe that they can hinder us on our path. Our motivation to ascend is to strengthen and purify ourselves in order to be stronger, purer instruments or channels, to be used in God's service. If in meditations, psychic experience spontaneously occur, we accept them as gifts to help guide us, but we do not use peyote, marijuana or anything other than our natural lifestyle (Yoga, Meditation, Diet, Selfless Service, etc.) to raise our vibration. We are encouraged to zone in our weak areas and work them. In our experience with spiritual aspirants, those who used drugs for many years, have a harder time than those who did not, as it did affect their physical, emotional or mental bodies. They also have a harder time with discipline, without which one cannot evolve. Evolution (ascension) requires hard work.

There are no fast, easy short-cuts. Drugs, even marijuana, is detrimental to the physical body.

Regeneration and Rejuvenation

The reconstruction and regeneration of the body is simpler than it would appear. It merely requires ample determination, patience, constant perseverance and time. Regeneration, becoming younger, is no mystic secret. It is common sense, but requires great self-discipline.

To become younger one has to attain health. To achieve a healthy physical body, requires knowing and understanding basic anatomy and physiology, in the same way that a mechanic knows and understands cars. To regenerate the body requires some basic knowledge and taking responsibility of one's own life and state of health, rather than resorting to the "quick fixes" so common on the market today.

Concentrated medicines and drugs may help to correct certain conditions, but only at the expense of damage to the same or other parts of the body at a future date. Most sick people are impatient to get quick, immediate results. It is easy to swallow a pill, get a shot or undergo an operation. Even the alternative medicines are frequently used as palliatives, without eradicating the root cause of the problem. Acupuncture, homeopathic remedies, Bach Flowers, if not administered correctly and if not used in conjunction with other necessary treatments, are prime examples. Society has been misinformed to resort to these remedies which require little effort or change of habits. Impatient for quick results, they do not realize that further complications could arise at a later date as a direct result of such remedies.

Nature takes time to heal and cure, but the results are permanent. If any part of the body is failing, one has to realize that all parts are interrelated, and the entire organism is involved. When Nature heals, the body is frequently subjected to reactions which must be endured with strength and patience, until Nature has finally reconstructed a healthier and younger body.

The human body is composed of trillions of microscopic cells, which in turn or composed of molecules and atoms. Each atom is a self-contained universe enclosing an enormous amount of energy and power. It is the life-principle in these atoms that makes it possible for each of us to possess a live, functioning body. This life-principle in the body is found in the form of enzymes. Enzymes are intangible, magnetic, Cosmic Energy. They activate substances and chemical reactions. Where there are enzymes, there is life. Enzymes are found in abundance in live food; they are destroyed when food is cooked.

The energy which enables all the parts of the body to operate, comes from the atoms composing them, together with the atoms composing the nutrition which they are fed i.e. the food we eat. Nutrition not only regenerates and rebuilds the cells and tissues of the physical body, but it is involved in the process of discarding waste matter from the body. The undigested food is eliminated from the body to prevent corruption in the form of fermentation and putrefaction in the body. If this putrefaction and corruption are allowed to accumulate in the body, it would be impossible to attain any degree of optimal health. If the type of food is correct and constructive, and waste matter is eliminated, the body responds by supplying an abundant amount of physical energy; the mind and emotions become balanced.

Life begets life. We cannot expect death to produce life. Thus the regeneration and replenishment of the life in our bodies must come from the life present in the food we eat. How do we eat life? Natural foods in their raw state contain life in the atoms and molecules composing them. This atomic life is referred to as enzymes. It is the enzymes which furnish the energy in the atoms found in the cells and tissues.

Organic food is food replete with enzymes and food which has been grown on balanced soil which has not been destroyed by chemical fertilizers. Organic food has been grown from unprocessed seed. The soil is full of earthworms as a result of proper composting and the complete absence of chemical fertilizers and poisonous sprays. All raw food is replete with enzymes but not all raw food is organically grown. Inorganic food is food which has been grown on nutrient deficient, toxic, unbalanced soil and it is food in which the enzymes have been destroyed by excessive heat.

The world's most serious problem is malnutrition. Civilized nations are as much afflicted with their abundance of foods, as nations who are lacking. Eat what tastes good, not what is nutritionally good for the body, seems to be the general attitude. To regenerate our bodies, we need to consume the highest quality organic food.

The fundamental purpose of eating is to replenish the chemical elements composing the cells and tissues in our body. Our physical body is a laboratory functioning under organic chemistry principles. Replenishment is one of the basic laws of Nature in regard to organic chemistry.

It is impossible to regenerate organic cells in a human body from inorganic (dead) matter. Inorganic food can sustain life but it cannot regenerate the cells and tissues of the body by supplying the chemical elements composing these. Dead cooked food sustains life at the expense of progressively degenerating health, energy and vitality. We need to replenish the body with food which is full of energy i.e. full of enzymes. All vegetables, fruits, nuts and seeds are, like the body, composed of billions of atoms. Every cell in the structure of these live foods, is endowed with live enzymes. Enzymes die at any temperature above 130 degrees Fahrenheit and are sensitive to heat above 118

53

degrees Fahrenheit. Cold, on the other hand, even sub-zero freezing, does not affect enzymes.

So both vegetation and the human body are composed of atomic elements. Both are live organisms whose atoms and cells abound in enzymes. The enzymes in the cells of the human body are exactly like those in vegetation. The atoms in the human body have a corresponding affinity for the like atoms in the vegetation ingested. Thus when certain atoms are needed to rebuild or replace body cells, there is a magnetic attraction which draws to such cells the exact kind and type of atomic elements needed for the work of replenishment or regeneration. This magnetic affinity occurs in the liver, which acts as a computer, and is directed by the functions of the endocrine glands. Combinations of atoms constitute chemical structures whose efficiency is dependent on the enzymes in the atoms of the vegetable cells just as much as on the enzymes of the body. Hence the need for an abundance of live food in the process of regeneration.

The endocrine glands are the laboratories of the human body. They generate ultramicroscopic substances called hormones. These hormones trickle directly into the bloodstream by the process of osmosis. It is the presence of enzymes throughout each gland that makes this transfer possible. The most important component of these hormones, besides their enzymes, is the number of rare and minute trace elements. Today it is known that the body is composed of 16 elements which compose the main structure of matter and 43 of these trace elements. Any lack or imbalance of any of these elements, is detrimental to health.

Vegetables are the builders of the body, containing a higher relative proportion of protein and a smaller proportion of carbon and carbohydrates. Fruits have a higher carbon (carbohydrate) content which serve to burn the toxins of the body, so they are the cleansers.

Every second of our existence, while there is life in the body, cells and tissues are being used up, and are miraculously replaced by new cells. These new cells can only be built from the material we put into our system – out of the atoms and molecules of the food we eat, the liquids we drink and the air we breathe.

The regeneration of the body requires energy. One has to learn how to generate and conserve energy. Energy consumers include: digestion of food; worry and negative thinking; excessive talking and socializing; overwork; living a self-centered, self-involved life. We have to learn the real joy of living. It is an art that requires overcoming every negative condition in our lives, by either changing the situation or removing yourself from it. All negative emotions such as worry, depression, fear, feelings of inferiority, have to be replaced with positive ones. The mind is never a blank – there are always either positive thoughts or negative ones. The way you feel in life – happy or otherwise indicates how positive or negative your thoughts are. There are so many thoughts that it's easier to gauge feelings than thoughts. Be aware of your feelings all the time and cleanse any negative emotions so that you are free to be out of yourself all the time and live for others, feeling, understanding and therefore loving them.

To conclude, vibrant health is the reflection of perfect harmony in all four bodies. Each microscopic cell of the body is endowed with life and intelligence. They respond to the stimulus of the mind, whether or not we are conscious of this. They are our servants and receive their programming directly from our minds. These servants need constant nourishment of the highest quality (good food and positive thoughts) in order to do their work. The quality of their work will be in direct proportion to the quality and quantity of the mind-food and physical food they are given. Overeating, even of the best food, creates toxicity of body and mind. It weakens the will and destroys the emotional body. Only eat what the body needs. You should always feel a little empty after a meal, never full. The mind should be clear and alert after a meal, never sluggish. If it's sluggish, you have overeaten. Most people do.

Health gained consciously through self-discipline, is rewarded by self-sufficiency and self-reliance, by strength. Regeneration and rejuvenation are more than feasible, but how many of us have the patience, determination, consistency and will-power that it demands? You could be one of the few.

Living The Greater Life

Introduction

Construct a strong, solid spiritual base that will enable you to weather any storm. Understand and then embrace the spiritual concepts in this little book. Live by them. Then focus on your service to the All and the world you have chosen, plus strengthening your mental body. Physical body disciplines are simply a must for a successful life. The physical body and spiritual body care are essential and have to be strong before you embark on strengthening the other bodies.

Service to the All is all you need to do to strengthen the emotional body. Your work for your world and studies will strengthen your mental body. Your personal emotional life will just naturally follow. It's not something you should or need to look for and try and make happen. Busy yourself with all the rest first, and this will naturally follow when the time is right.

Be happy in life no matter what. Let this be your eternal life goal. Be happy no matter who you are with or not with, where you are or aren't etc. Cherish life. Value it. Appreciate and enjoy every moment, and put your all into it. Your life attitude is everything. It is what will pervade all you do, making it hugely successful or otherwise.

Live to love and you will enter the Greater Life, a life of joy in service to the God of the All and His Creation.

The Perfection of the Cosmic Order

- ❖ The perfection of the Cosmic Order will always reign supreme.
- ❖ The Cosmic Order is perfect. All is in order in the Cosmos, even if it appears not to be so after this disastrous negative era that went so evil. The perfection of the Cosmic order can be grasped by studying the sciences and through direct experience, by living a spiritual life.
- ❖ There is Divine Justice in the Cosmos that never errs. If a person's heart is in the right place, no matter what happens to him/her, s/he will always be taken care of by the Cosmos. (Therefore never worry about what will happen to you or loved ones. Worry about getting your heart in the right place in life, and keeping it there).
- ❖ Excessive negative is evil and even this was allowed in the Cosmic Order because man had to learn what evil could do. Evil – the hunger for power, beauty, position, possessions; and jealousy and greed, borne from the desire for one or usually all of these things, transforms people and actions into evil.
- ❖ By the Cosmic energetic Law of Rhythm, as evil as everything went, it will now go excessively positive.

58

Purity of Heart is Everything

- Service to the God of the All is where one's heart should always reside. Serve Him by serving your world and universe and the people in your life.
- Start every day with an expression of gratitude to the God of the All. Your service to the Cosmos, the Divine Father of the All, should be your greatest joy in life.
- A person's heart cannot be touched. You can destroy someone physically and mentally, but they will just shut down after a certain point and enter an unconscious state. You cannot touch a person's emotional or spiritual bodies, if they are strong.
- Love is not everything. Purity of heart is everything.

Relationships - Loved Ones

- The more perfect your relationship regardless of the dimension, the stronger your love bond, the higher your level of connection (communication), the less likely you are to lose loved ones.
- Have the greatest faith in the Cosmic Order and surrender your loved ones to its care if and when necessary.
- If a union is so perfect (spouse, child, parent, friend, God), it will be irreplaceable, and you will therefore always be together. The bond can never be severed and never will. Accept the Cosmic Order and temporary separation if it ever occurs but know that you will be together forever. Accept the Cosmic Order with obedience and comprehension that everything is perfect and for

the best, and know that deep love bonds can and never will be broken.

❖ Anything that is so perfect in life, endures. The more perfect the love bond, the more impossible it is to break. It will endure and survive, no matter how tsunamic the storm of life. Things and relationships that are imperfect, do not endure.

❖ Don't get attached to people and situations. Just do your very best in every situation and with the people in your life currently and your life will always be so beautiful, so perfect.

❖ There are relationships and eternal relationships. Your eternal relationships are the strong, perfect ones that will endure for all eternity and you can therefore be attached to them but know that dimensional separation is a possibility. However, one day all eternal relationships will be united and never separated, in heaven.

Let Service in Life be your Joy

❖ Live for the greatest. Dedicate your life to the greatest and you'll always be happy in life.

❖ Just learn to get the right guidance in life and follow it. It will lead you to purify and strengthen yourself and others. Herein lies your eternal happiness.

❖ Don't limit yourself to anything that is human, not even the most perfect relationships. Cherish and value them but never make them your everything. Your everything must be your service to the God of the All and His Divine Plan.

❖ Come through with your life disciplines, focusing on those that are most difficult for you, in order to serve the Cosmos to the best of your ability.

- ❖ Rise above the human drama in your service. Your happiness has to lie in this service more than in any personal relationships, as much as you must love and cherish these relationships.
- ❖ Guiding children in life, as a parent or teacher, is a sacred job. Strengthen and purify yourself so that you are worthy of the job and perform it well. You affect a child's entire eternal evolution either positively or negatively, depending on who you are as a person because a child will learn from and follow your example, rather than your words.
- ❖ Heart and mind focus are everything. The success of your service and plenitude you live in life, will be in direct proportion to your mind and heart focus in each life activity.
- ❖ Purify and strengthen yourself through your disciplines and through loving extensively and expansively. Become a strong pure channel for your service to the All.
- ❖ There is a God of the All and that is the constant in your life that you are meant to hold onto. Live to serve Him by serving his through service to your world. We each choose a world which corresponds to our level of consciousness. If you chose your world, value it and serve it to ensure its survival.
- ❖ Have faith and allow the Cosmos to use you as it needs.

The Connection

❖ A strong connection to an evolved soul on a higher dimension is an essential life tool.

❖ Learn to connect to your guide, God, Jesus or anyone you feel close to and want to be guided by.

❖ Connections are like muscles – be it a connection with someone on your dimension or from a higher dimension. The more a connection is used, the stronger you make it. You create an energy that cannot be severed. Each connection has a strength level.

❖ Be receptive to guidance in life. We are constantly being guided but are too active and busy to realize it. Be guided by a child's remark, a bird's flight, the sunset and cloud formation. Keep yourself good and strong in life so that you are free to be receptive and guided. Listen to life's guidance attentively.

❖ A high level connection is the greatest gift you can ever have because you'll always be guided in life and you'll never lose loved ones.

❖ To attain a high level connection requires mastering Chakras 1 to 6. Anyone can do it if it's what you want.

❖ A union of souls through love bonds, on the same dimension or across dimensions, creates a force. A union of two souls results in double force – the sum total of the force of both people. A union of three souls results in triple force etc. Shatter your ego in order to be able to connect to others who share your service to the world and All life goals. In this way an indomitable body of force will be created.